I0027177

Men, the Movement:

Let's Help Them

Men, the Movement:
Let's Help Them

**Written & Created by Michelle Swogger
and the J Team**

Illustrated by Melina Mangino

Men, the Movement: Let's Help Them

Written & Created by Michelle Swogger and the J Team

Doc Publishing
2025

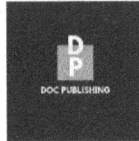

Copyright © 2025 by Michelle Swogger

All rights reserved. This book or any portion thereof may not be reproduced or used in any manner whatsoever without the express written permission of the publisher except for the use of brief quotations in a book review or scholarly journal.

First Printing: 2025

ISBN: 978-1-7358559-3-6

Doc Publishing
P.O. Box 7503
New Castle, PA 16107

www.docpublishing.org

Dedication

A special thank you to my fabulous husband, sons, brothers-in-law, sister-in-law, nephews, nieces and the rest of the family for teaching me the true meaning of family. I love you all.

Also, a special acknowledgement must go to my spiritual writers, the J Team. Thanks for the walks and talks.

Sincerely,

Michelle Swogger

A few words from the Author

This book is written in support of all the men in this world who feel muted by the pressures from society. The stories may be fictional but please understand that **Andropause is a very real condition.** Equality is of the utmost importance in women's rights, there is little debate on that. But in my eyes, equality must also mean the equality of men's rights and abilities to express fear, sadness, anxiety, the whole spectrum in the world of emotion.

We, as women, often focus on our own strengths and needs and that is rightfully so. But we also need to reach out and lend a helping hand to our brothers, sons, friends, husbands, etc. Women and men are both strong. We are all allowed to feel weak at times. I don't think everyone knows that.

It is a reflection of what could be very real situations and experiences that men could go through in their lives. They are symbolic of daily struggles that men sometimes face often alone, with no support or guidance. My goal is to gently enlighten those who may be going through similar situations, and let them know it's ok to reach out and ask for help.

I chose the title "Men, the Movement" because my goal is for the book to do just that. Create a movement toward finding help, expand medical research, and perhaps more importantly, move all of us to have compassion, knowledge and understanding when we see our male loved ones, friends or neighbors going through things that sometimes make them feel like strangers to us.

The story is told through the lens of the main character, Mrs. R., a loving mother, neighbor, and teacher with a mission to start a movement.

From this amateur's desk, I present you with Men, the Movement.

Table of Contents

Introduction

She was so perplexed. As she sat on her back porch, gliding and watching the animals in the yard, seeing the hummingbirds hover over the sweet nectar of the flowers she planted, she couldn't help thinking back on a conversation she recently had with one of her best friends.

She just couldn't believe what was happening. It seems like she hears the same story over and over these days. The story of friends and how they are struggling. How can a person be sitting in an environment like hers and not be able to enjoy the birds, the weather, the beauty of the day? It's like an epidemic that husbands, brothers, sons and fathers seem to be going through. She wondered what she could do about this hidden society.

Hidden not by choice, but perhaps because those who are in this struggling group do not know how to be seen and those not in the group don't know what to look for.

Now, this woman was no stranger to any society. In fact, she was quite well known as the Health and Home Economics teacher at the local middle school. Her name was Anna but her students fondly called her Mrs. R. She was loved by all who knew her and she felt the same way about everyone she met. Mrs. R. only saw the good in everyone and had compassion for those she saw struggling in life.

It was with all that compassion that she noticed this pattern. This health crisis affects men of different ages and lifestyles. Of course she saw all the other health issues affecting men, women, and children, but this is a condition that she doesn't remember hearing much about at all. As a mother of four boys herself, and the wife of a man that can be quite mysterious at times, this pattern quickly became vitally important to her.

Mrs. R. loved to write. She felt that if she could write a series of short stories similar to the ones she had been hearing about and group them together, maybe a pattern would form or someone would learn something that could help this hidden society of suffering men.

With a simple notepad and pen, she started on her journey. Not only did she hope that these stories could raise awareness and show the need for more research on men's mental health, but she also thought they may help those going through such troubling times.

Now, Mrs. R. was a simple, humble, wonderful woman. She never saw herself as a professional writer, but she wanted to try. She thought of each story that her friends had shared with her and developed make-believe characters who encountered similar issues in their make-believe lives. "Hmm short stories, that's kinda boring," Mrs. R. thought. "I want to call them books. Tiny Books," fondly named after the first character, Tiny.

Book 1, Tiny

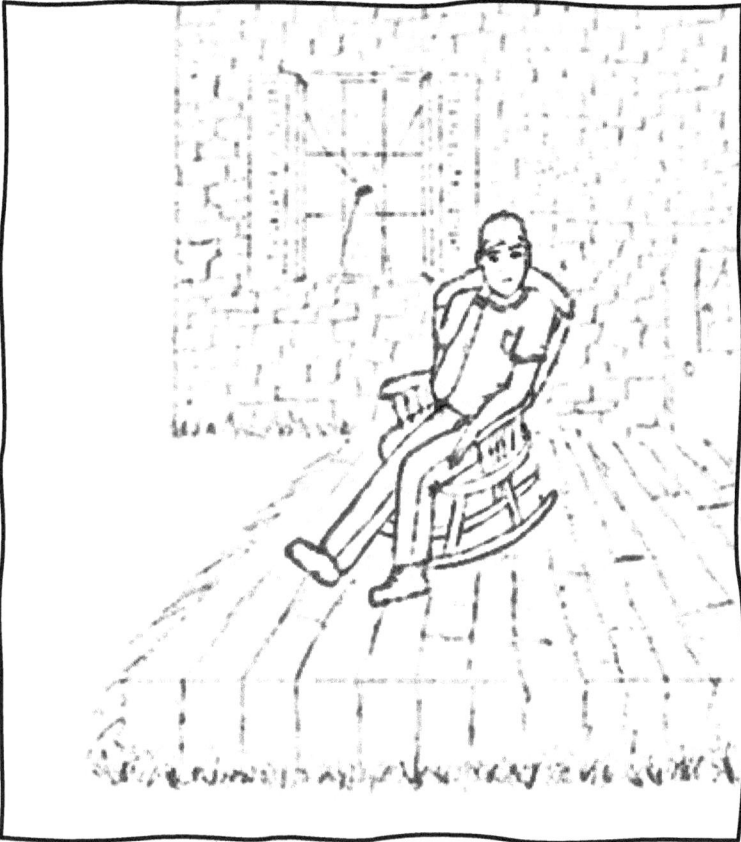

Once upon a time there was a boy named

Tiny. Tiny was in one word, unstoppable. From

his first LOUD breath, there was nothing small

about Tiny. His strong, dynamic and constant

aura of happiness, confidence and compassion made him a magnet. Everyone wanted to be around Tiny. Did other kids make fun of his name? Sometimes, but Tiny would just smile, laugh and say, "That was a good one." He wasn't bothered with things like that.

When Tiny was old enough for school, his home quickly became the neighborhood hang out. On any given day after school, his big yard would have two teams of kids playing games and sports. Football, baseball, tag, kick ball, you name it, Tiny's yard was always a sports field. The kids who didn't want to play just hung out to be with the cool kids that knew Tiny. They also knew that they were always welcome to go into Tiny's house for food, snacks and drinks. His house was always filled with the aroma of something delicious floating in the air.

In Tiny's world all kids were cool kids. Tiny had no enemies. He just loved and saw value in everyone. Tiny enjoyed school. He was good with his grades and liked almost all the subjects. When high school came, he was on top of it all. He played sports, went to all the dances and graduated at the top of his class.

Tiny went on to breeze through college and had a full-time job to help with his family's expenses. When stresses in life became challenging, Tiny seemed stronger than all of them. He never had a bad day. A forever optimist, Tiny never gave up his positive attitude and zest for life. After college Tiny snagged a management level job, got his first car and even got engaged.

Life was easy and breezy.

Before Tiny knew it, there were two kids laughing and playing in the yard of his first home. Those kids from his old neighborhood now drove to his house and brought their families for get-togethers and bonfires.

Through time there were growing kids, job transfers, promotions and moves. Even though life was going in the right direction, one morning Tiny woke up and didn't seem to feel quite as unstoppable as he did before. Nothing was much different in his life. The kids were doing well, his wife was fine, things were smooth, just as smooth as ever, but Tiny noticed he just didn't have the zest that he used to. He shrugged it off and went on about his daily routine. He would shake it, he thought.

But he didn't. Now in his mid-50s the things that never used to get to Tiny, started bothering him now. The language from his childhood friends also started changing when they would talk. Instead of talking about pretty girls, cars and sports, the dialogue centered on bills, ailments and home improvements that few could really afford.

At work, the demand seemed to have a higher stress level than before. He started focusing on the possible consequences if his job performance should slow instead of striving for the next job promotion.

At this point, Tiny started dreading every morning. His focus shifted from all that was right in his world to all that could go wrong in his world. His demands at work changed a bit and instead of going with the flow, he started feeling foggy. The tasks that he used to breeze through suddenly became almost impossible to do. He just didn't feel like himself anymore. He went from feeling like a king to a coward and was afraid he was letting everyone down. No one else felt that way, but he did.

Tiny had lost his will to live and began wondering if life was even worth living anymore. There were times when he actually considered taking his own life. Yet no one knew how troubled he was.

He went to several doctors and was told repeatedly, "Oh you are just stressed, you need yoga." Why don't you play golf more?" "Do you meditate?" "Here are some meds. These will mute the stressors. Watch out for the side effects though, and you could get addicted, and they may even make you feel worse. Best of luck to you."

Nothing worked. And by the way, Tiny didn't like yoga. Yoga would make him even more stressed. Tiny wasn't into the traditional meditation, sound bowling and reiki lifestyle. Tiny was a jock, an amazing scholar, father and husband but who was he? He didn't know. Where did Tiny go?

Really? Mrs. R. went over her story. Her Tiny Book. It was her very first one. "Poor Tiny," she thought, "I just wish there was something we could do to help these men." It made her think, if there was more research, more information, more awareness on these mystery issues, how would that change Tiny's outcomes? She took that thought and ran with it. For the rest of the Tiny books, she wrote a Part 1 and called it, "The Struggle" and a Part 2 called "The Wish." To make each story feel complete, she even added the words "The End" so that each tiny book felt complete. She started with John.

Book 2, John

Part 1, The Struggle

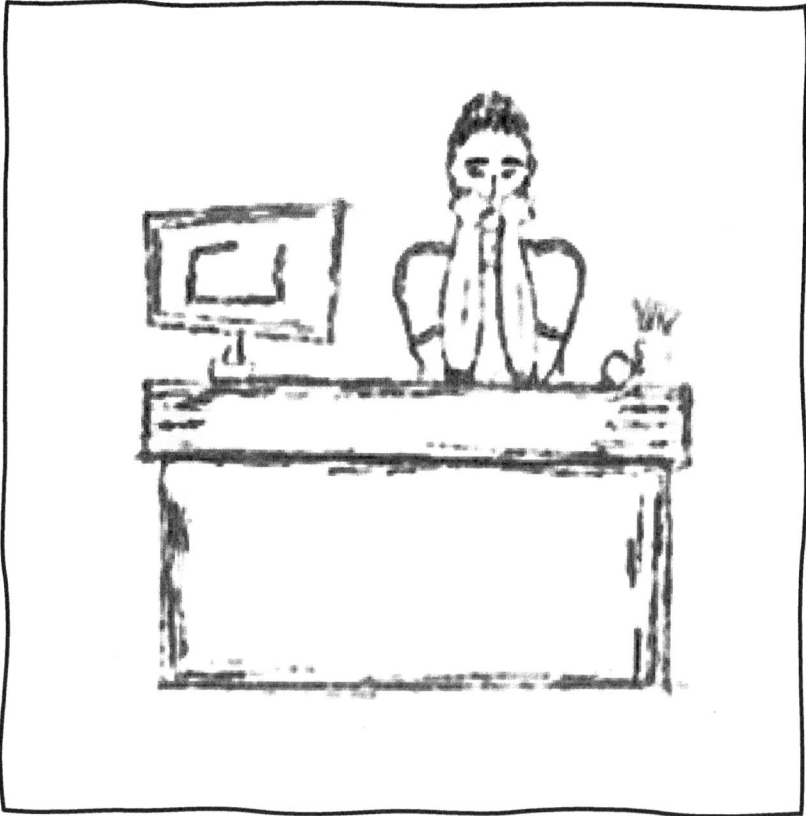

Once upon a time there was a man named

John. John was a young strong man looking for

work. One day he walked into a local warehouse

and applied for any available position he could get. He was interested in making money so he could live his fullest life.

A little green behind the ears, John's goal was to work hard and play hard. He didn't really care what he did for work and he wasn't afraid of physical labor. John loved coming home with a tired body. It seemed to empower his mind. He loved using the muscles that he was built with and making the most of all he was given. To him, a few calluses, stiff muscles, cuts and bruises just meant he had earned his pay.

At night John enjoyed relaxing with his wife, sitting by a fire and dreaming of a long future, maybe a kid or two, a family pet. The sky was the limit.

John made no mistake walking into that warehouse. He ended up walking into that same warehouse for over 20 years. The more experience he got, the more promotions he received.

His job became a little less physically demanding, which was okay with his aging body. He still enjoyed having those sore muscles, but he liked that they came from backyard football with his kids, rather than a long day at work.

Finally, he was able to save enough money and get that bigger house they needed as well as reliable cars for the family to enjoy.

John was a simple man leading a wholesome life. One day he walked into work and noticed a buzz amongst his staff. He asked, "Why all the chatter today?" "Oh, you didn't hear?"

asked a coworker. "They are shutting us down. It's going to be bad." John just smiled and said, "Okay, if I had a nickel for every time I heard a rumor like that..." and he went on about his day. This time the rumors didn't stop. In fact, information validating what that coworker had said started coming in from those who were higher up in the company.

One fateful day, after 20 years with a company he had grown to love, John was given notice that he was being let go but not without a nice severance package.

John was sad and disappointed at first. He was losing a whole family—his work family. He knew he wanted to go right back into the workforce and hopefully find a new work family.

With his skill set, it didn't take long for John to get hired at another company. It all started great. Even though he missed his old job, his old routine and of course his friends, he was confident that he would settle in at this new place. But there were differences.

This job had a different, more distant feel with the staff. For one thing John was older than most of them. The ethics were different. Not better or worse, just different. Soon it became like oil and water and he just couldn't fit in.

He tried another workplace. He soon had the same feelings as he did at the first one he tried. John, who once fit like a glove in the workforce, started feeling like a misfit everywhere. He couldn't cope with newer technology and more modern atmospheres. John felt as if he had aged out. He tried job after job. His reactions to the jobs and his inability to cope with all the changes got worse in his mind. He just didn't know how to live outside his old workplace. His mindset started affecting everything. He soon lost his zest to enjoy his wife and his kids. He didn't care about his hobbies anymore. John had lost his will to live. As his wife and family looked on, it begged the question, where did John go?

Mrs. R. read John's story again. "I wish," she thought, "That I could create a world in which John wouldn't have been so blindsided by everything happening to him. His job, his feelings, everything." And then, she thought of a whole other world for John. One that would not only help him, but others who worked for that same company.

Part 2, The Wish

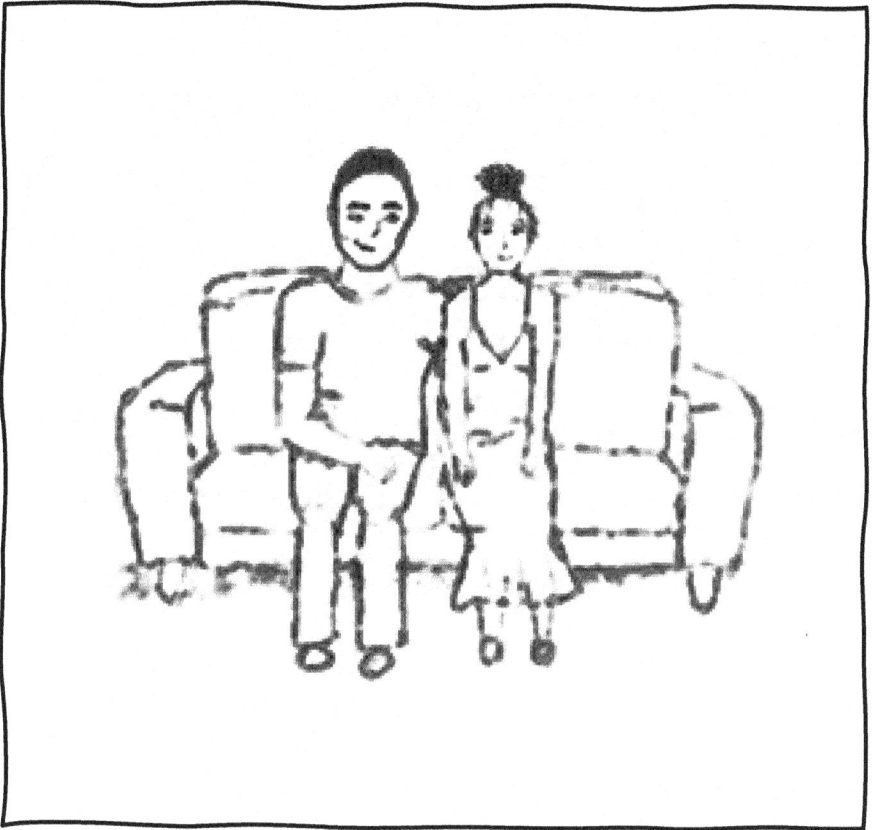

Fortunately for John and the rest of the

employees, the company did extensive research

on the possible effects that the news may have

on employees. They incorporated a three-step program.

1. The employees were notified further in advance than before so that everyone would have plenty of time to make necessary adjustments in their lives.

2. As part of the severance package, the company hired counselors who specialize in the mental health effects that this may have on the employees and offered their services before, during and up to one year after employment, which included weekly in-house visits from their appointed counselor.

3. Employees were provided resources from the local career program that offers job training, help with resume writing, applying

for unemployment benefits and various other valuable resources.

John was scared and overwhelmed at first, but with the tools provided by the company, he was able to secure a new job and get the emotional help he needed any time he started to feel overwhelmed. Now, John feels like John again.

The End

Mrs. R. loved thinking of ways to make these characters come back to life, so she continued with her "Wish" stories. She thought of a story about a boy named Tom.

Book 3, Tom

Part 1, The Struggle

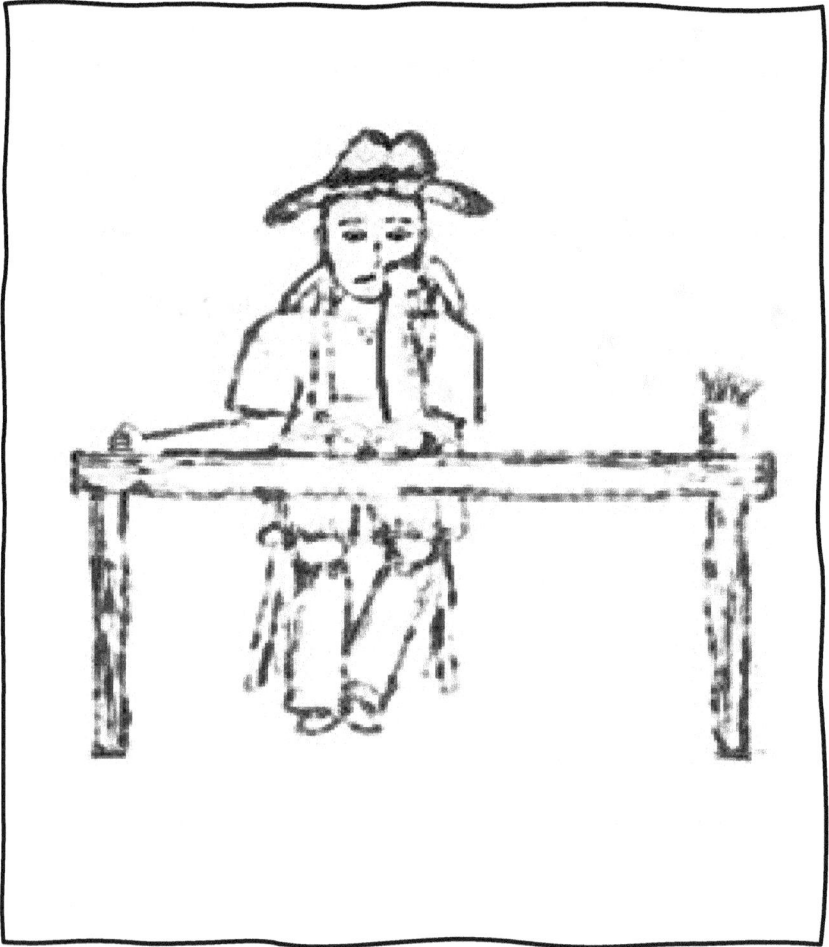

Once upon a time, a long time ago there

was a young boy named Tom. Tom lived deep in

the Rocky Mountains. Mountain living was a very rough way of life especially in the times before cars, plumbing and electricity. You had to love the land if you wanted to feel happy. Tom felt happy. He didn't know of any other way to live but he didn't need to. He woke up every day with a heart filled with love, adventure and passion for his little log home that his dad built, the food that his family grew, harvested and lived from and of course the nature that surrounded him.

From the good to the scary, he loved it all. From the eagles soaring high in the sky to the fog nestling itself between the mountain peaks in the morning. Even the mysterious but wondrous sounds of all things that lurked in the darkness every night, Tom knew he was surrounded with life's truest wealth.

His family had a horse and a wagon and on occasion they would travel down the mountain to go to the local store. If Tom was lucky, he would have earned a penny or two to buy his favorite candy. That made life even more enjoyable for him.

Tom and his mother, father, brothers and sisters lived off the land. They earned money from selling herbs from the forest and animal hide. Almost every day there were visits from friends and family from near and far who enjoyed sitting on the porch, looking out on the land and exchanging news, family stories and a lot of laughter. He spent his young days listening to his elders and learning of the trials and tribulations they had endured.

On occasion some of the visitors brought banjos, fiddles and harmonicas and sang the songs of the mountains. True stories, but to music. A person can learn a lot from those songs. He listened to the words of all the songs that had been written about their way of life. It seems in those days, their best form of therapy was through the written word, put to music. From the words to the tone of each song, whether happy or soulful, most songs seemed like a cry for help, or a celebration of joy to be shared by all who would listen.

As Tom got older, he decided that he wanted to find a way to share all this love with others who weren't as rich as him. Tom started writing about all he had seen, all he knew, and all he learned about the land and his life on that mountain.

At the local store he saw an advertisement in the local paper. The ad said that the newspaper was looking for local stories to publish. Tom used his money to buy that paper instead of candy. As soon as he got home, he got one of his stories ready and sent it to the paper in the hopes that it would be chosen. It sure was! As fast as lightning, and lightning is fast, a career was born. Tom's Tales became sought after across the nation. This is exactly what Tom wanted.

Now in his 40s, he spent years writing books and stories much to the delight of all who read them. They were a demanding group of followers. They wanted more and more. At first this was wonderful but as time passed, the passion became replaced with pressure. Pressure to think of new stories, pressure of timelines. He had to write so much that he couldn't get out and enjoy all that he himself loved about his life.

Tom's mindset started to shift. He went from waking up happy and full of life to waking up tired, stressed and full of pressure and deadlines. All his dreams had come true. He was living his best life, but he never felt worse.

These new feelings caused a panic in Tom. He couldn't think clearly anymore. He couldn't observe the very things that he lived to write about. Tom didn't even feel like himself anymore. His life didn't feel like his life anymore. He stood on the front porch of his home, staring at the mountains as if it were a foreign country. He asked himself, Who am I? Where am I? Why do I feel dead? What if I was dead? Maybe my family would be better off?" Where did Tom go?

"Okay Tom," Mrs. R. thought. "Life has somehow blinded you from all that you love. Let's see if we can find a way to take those blinders off. What if your story went a little like this?"

Part 2, The Wish

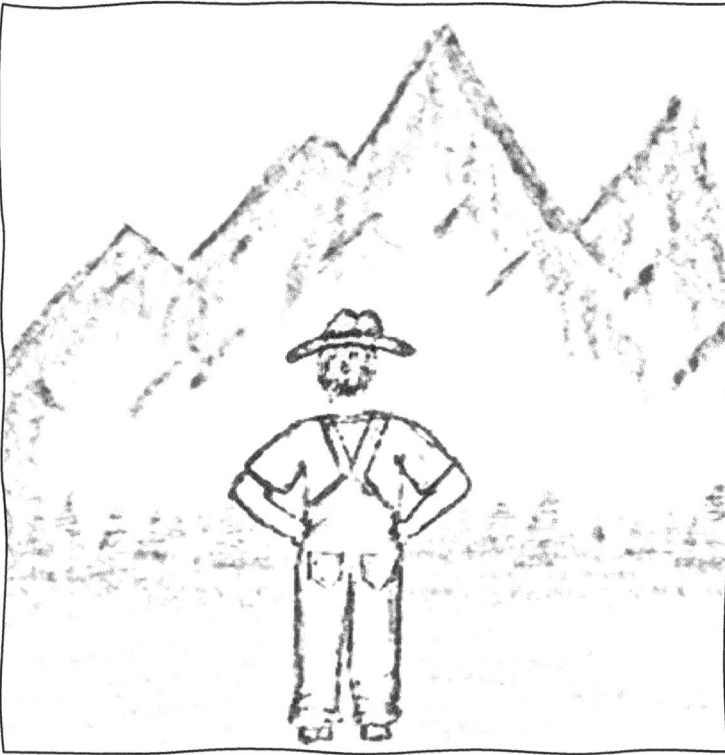

Somewhere along Tom's crazy winding

road, Tom ran into another scholar of sorts. One

who studied the mind and the effects that life can

have on it. He gave Tom some great advice. He

said, "Son, pay attention to the stories about

YOUR life. When you start to feel strange, talk to

someone who deals with the mind like me,
BEFORE those stories start to snowball in your
head. We can help."

Tom went right back to the very paper
where he saw the ad for stories. In that paper he
found an ad for "The Moodologist." That was the
name this psychologist went by. Tom liked the
unique name enough that he wrote a letter and
reached out to him. Several letters back and forth
led Tom to seek some other tests from his
physician as well as learning coping skills to help
when his mind started racing. Priority one: Stop
all of it and get back into nature until you feel
better. The world will wait.

The End

"Wow", Mrs. R. thought, "If only life were this easy to change." It could be if people just knew more about what our poor fellows are feeling. Her friends also shared with her that when one member is not feeling right, the whole family feels it as well. That made her think of her next story about a mom named Martha.

Book 4, Martha

Part 1, The Struggle

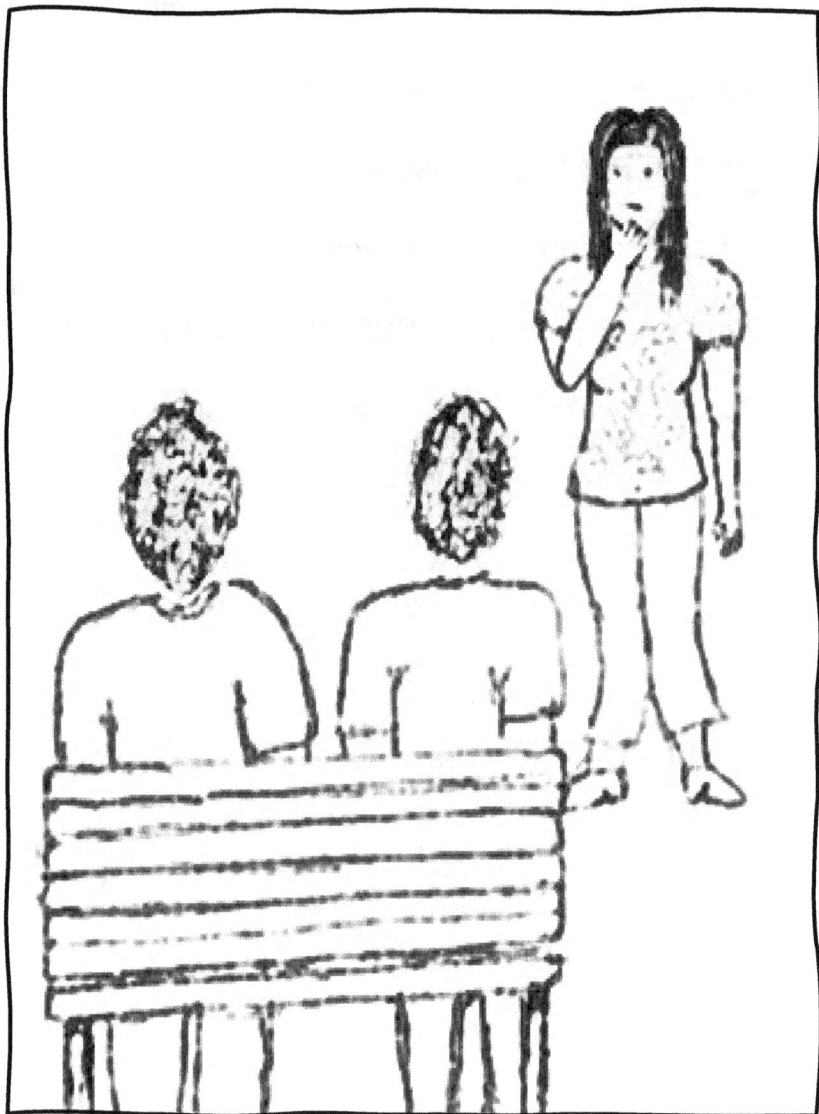

Once upon a time there was a woman named Martha. There was a time when you couldn't wipe the smile from Martha's face. The one thing she had always wanted had finally come true. Martha and her husband were expecting their first child. It was a glorious time for them. They eagerly decorated the nursery and traded their coupe for a minivan. Their friends hosted a baby shower and after nine months, Martha gave birth to a healthy baby boy. She was financially able to be a stay-at-home mom and loved every second of it. She loved it so much that in a couple of years they did it all over again. Two happy baby boys!

Martha soon realized that everyone was right when they said time goes so fast. It seemed like in the blink of an eye Martha was at her oldest son's college graduation. This was a man who was so bright that he didn't know what getting a B on a report card felt like. He constantly and consistently excelled at all that was put before him. Even though the world saw that as nothing short of miraculous, Martha saw the toll that it truly took on her son. The pressure that he constantly put himself under was so overwhelming that he started having medical issues such as stomach problems, panic attacks and constant stress. This was such a change from her youngest son who seemed to be blessed with more of a life balance than her first.

Her younger son simply didn't sweat the small stuff. In fact, he really didn't sweat much stuff at all. In his opinion, life is going to happen so enjoy what you can and don't worry about the rest. That was until he went into puberty. His mind and body were not corresponding with each other. This internal fight caused stress and paralyzing anxiety.

There is nothing more painful than seeing a child suffer. When her oldest son was a child, Martha was able to help, somewhat, during the times he became stressed, but as he got older and moved away, she lost her ability to help in the ways she used to. A stuffed animal or fun trip to the park lost its healing powers after a while.

Her son went to doctor after doctor but always came back with only a few answers. By now, the younger brother had overcome what he was going through and, in a way, became a source of comfort and healing for the whole family. A true testament to family values.

Martha learned that she wasn't alone in having a son struggle with anxiety and breakdowns. Other moms shared with Martha that they too have had to stand by helplessly as they watch their sons struggle with those same crippling mental breakdowns. It seemed all of them were met with the same results: medication and prescribed diet changes. Of the mom's she knew, there was never an "AHA" moment to identify what was going on. They often thought to themselves, "Where did our boys go?"

"Oh Martha, let's get your family back on track! I am going to turn this all around!" thought Mrs. R.

Part 2, The Wish

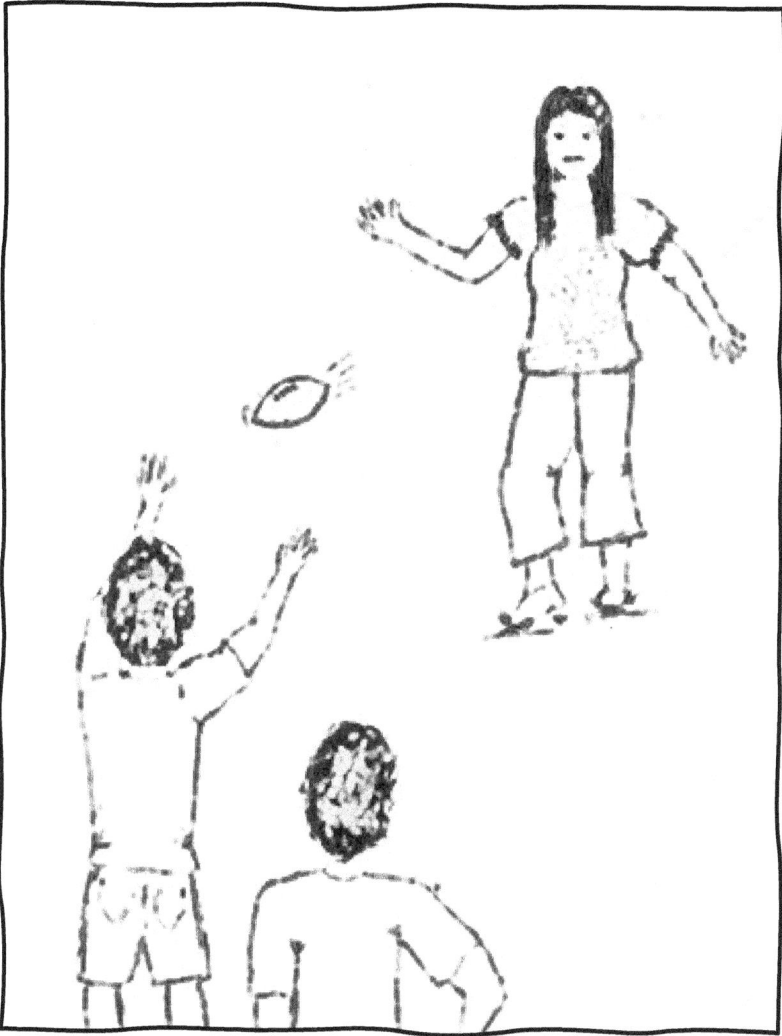

Martha's family lived near some of the most

world class medical centers. It seemed that the

typical treatments weren't working as well as she had hoped. When she was talking with one of the other parents in her community, the parent asked "Have you tried a more holistic approach? My kids were having similar issues as yours and I found a doctor who specializes in more holistic techniques. It really made a difference."

Martha was willing to try something different. She and her kids made the change and it made all the difference in the world. The doctor worked with each child individually and researched each symptom they were having. Soon the boys were thriving again. This doctor even noted that kids who have higher anxiety levels may experience more serious midlife changes as men. She wanted Martha to be mindful of that.

The End

Mrs. R. found writing these stories, these

Tiny books, quite emotionally cleansing to her.

She tried to write a variety of scenarios so that

others may find one with which they could relate.

She continued with Carnell.

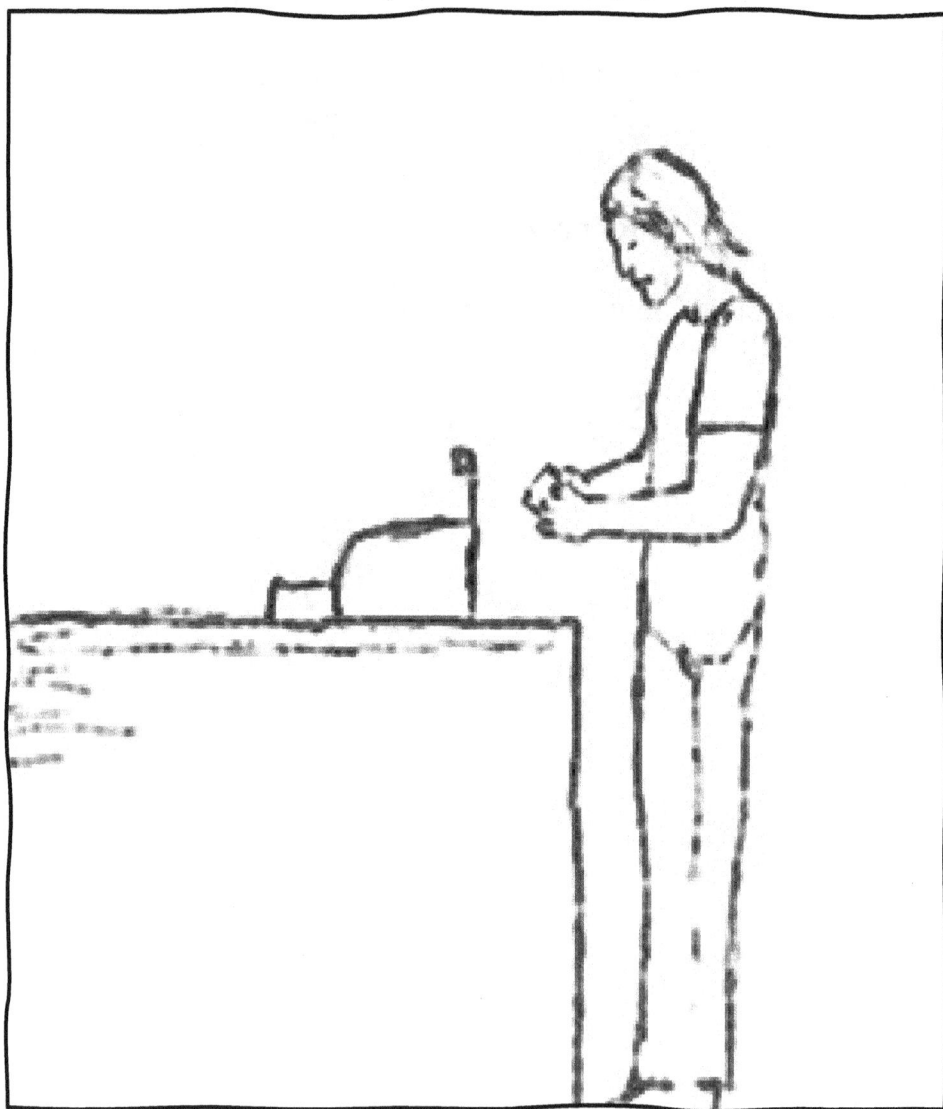

Book 5, Carnell

Part 1, The Struggle

Once upon a time there was a man named Carnell. Carnell was a single man working two jobs: his career, and his fun job at a local pet store. He loved his career in the medical field but his job at the pet store was just plain fun. His life was truly in perfect alignment. Career, fun job, family and friends, things were great.

One day at the pet shop the manager got a call from Carnell. He wasn't feeling well and had to call off. Carnell was normally very healthy but everyone has a down day once in a while so the manager didn't think much of it. The next weekend came along. The manager got another call. Carnell couldn't come in. This went on for over two months.

Finally, Carnell had to admit that he was experiencing extreme depression and anxiety. He was getting help but needed time. Because Carnell was such a wonderful employee, the pet store covered his hours until he could come back. Nothing in Carnell's life had changed. But his reactions to his life changed. He said he felt as if he was trapped in a deep dark tunnel with no way out. At first, he thought he would shrug it off as just a bad day. But it was too big for him. He couldn't fight it. The prison that he found himself in daily started affecting both of his jobs. He lost his ability to go to either job. He even stopped calling them to let them know.

He knew this was not like him at all. He started wondering who he really was, as he felt he was a stranger to himself. He would walk around his home thinking and wondering "Where did I go?"

"Carnell, it's time for you to get back to

YOU." Mrs. R knew Carnell could get back to his

old self with a few changes here and there.

Part 2, The Wish

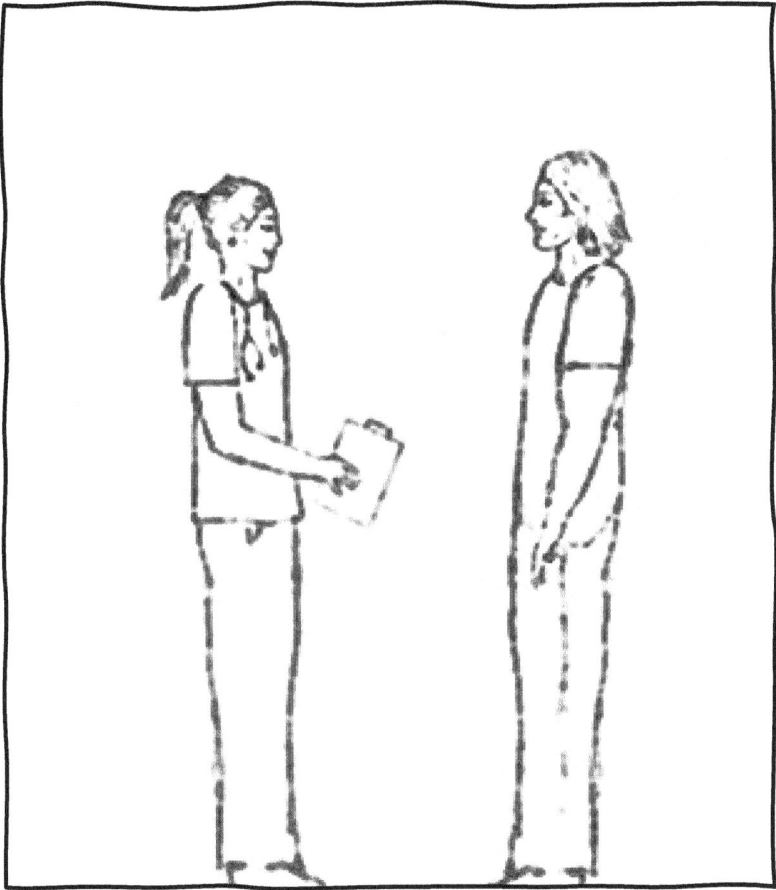

Carnell had finally had enough of feeling like this. In his late 30's he finally decided to go to his doctor. The doctor ordered what seemed to be every test imaginable, from head scans, to MRIs to stress tests. He also ran a series of tests that measured a man's hormone levels. This was a fairly new approach to the medical field and one that is usually ordered for middle aged women.

After carefully reviewing each result, the doctor determined Carnell was in a pre-midlife crisis. "Ok, what the heck is midlife? Isn't that a woman thing?" asked Carnell. The doctor chuckled. "It's more common than you think. The medical industry has been doing more and more research on the mental complications men sometimes go through as they age. So, let's work together to prepare you for this because it's the start of several changes that some men go

through. But relax, we have treatments and

answers. You did the right thing by coming in."

The End

"I'm glad I got Carnell straightened out.

Now what about poor Carl?", thought Mrs. R.

Let's see what we can do for him.

Book 6, Carl

Part 1, The Struggle

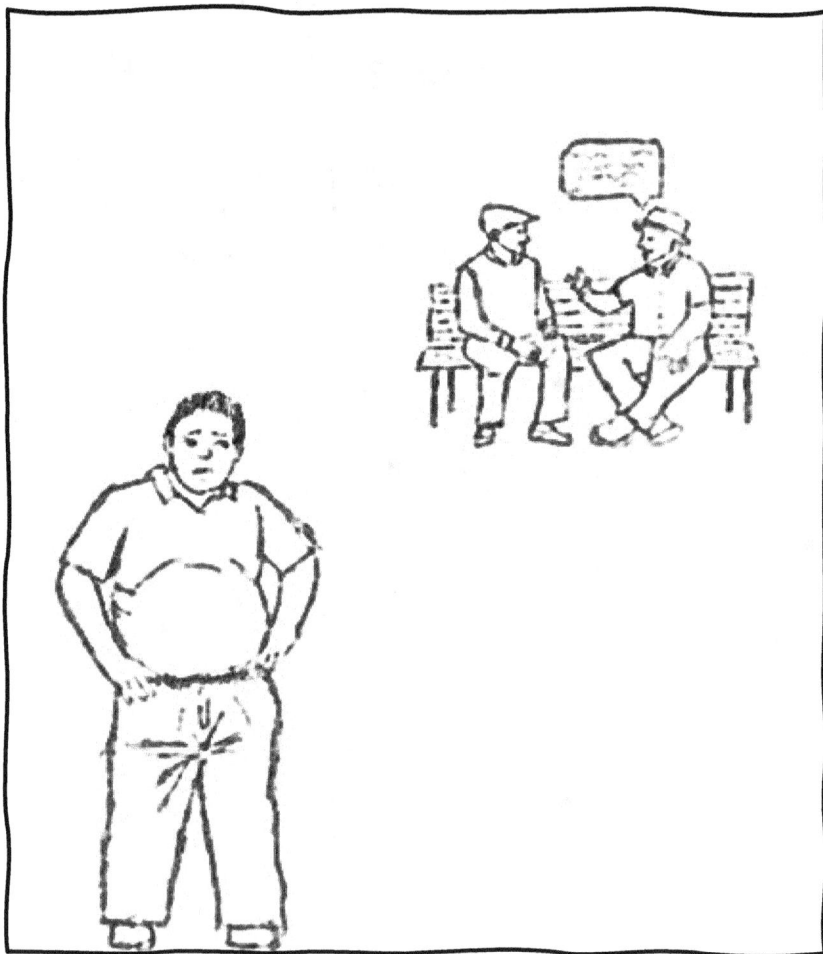

Once upon a time there was a man named Carl. Carl was entering into the sunset of his life. He had worked for over 40 years, raised a family and been happily married to the love of his life for years. Carl did it. He had reached the point where that magic word became reality--RETIREMENT.

Carl had been planning for years for this moment in his life. Oh, the fishing he was going to do! He had his car to restore and his winemaking was sure to flourish. Ahhh the beauty of time given to him after a well-earned career.

At first that's how it felt. No more early mornings. Carl could wake up, enjoy his coffee with his wife, and decide what to do with all that time. It felt like the dream vacation. He had complete control over his time.

For a while, Carl still felt young and vibrant. He caught up on home projects. He cleaned the cars. The yard never looked better.

One Saturday he went to the auto store and ran into some of his former co-workers who were still in the workforce. He smiled and greeted them with joy. They greeted him in quite the same way. They were very happy to see him. After they exchanged some quick conversations, Carl went on to look for the parts he needed. As he shopped, he couldn't help overhearing them talking. It was shop talk about work. As Carl listened, he realized he couldn't relate to what they were talking about. He didn't recognize names and the terms they were using were different. He walked back over to them and joined in once again on the conversation. He said "Hey I heard you talking about the plant, how are things there?" One of them politely answered, "Oh yeah, same old same old." They each went on to their own shopping.

That was when it first hit Carl. He felt so odd. He felt obsolete. He had heard them talking about new things happening, but when he tried to be a part of the conversation, it was clear he no longer fit in. He used to matter every day at that plant. Now, it's as if he never worked there. That is quite hard emotionally. He felt... old. Outdated. He shrugged it off and just went on about his "happy" retirement.

But a little seed had been planted that day at the parts store. A seed of uselessness and unimportance. That seed started growing each day and before he knew it, instead of focusing on all the fun things he can do with all his time, his mindset shifted toward feeling that his time had no value. Without work, who was Carl? Carl was old, outdated and discarded. His wife saw the change in Carl's attitude and did all she could to help him see his value now as a retired man. But Carl's work had become his identity for almost fifty years.

It was like a wave came over him. Each day, instead of getting up in the morning, enjoying coffee and casual conversation with his wife, he stopped wanting to get out of bed. The things he thought he would do, fishing, hunting, enjoying time with friends, became unimportant to him. He went from feeling like he had finally made it and was on top of the world, to feeling rejected, kicked to the curb and worthless. His loved ones didn't even recognize him anymore. The man they had counted on for years was crumbling right before their eyes with no apparent reason as to why. After a while, Carl didn't even recognize himself. He looked at a stranger when he looked in the mirror. Where did Carl go?

"Carl," Mrs. R. thought, "Let me make those retirement dreams come true."

Part 2, The Wish

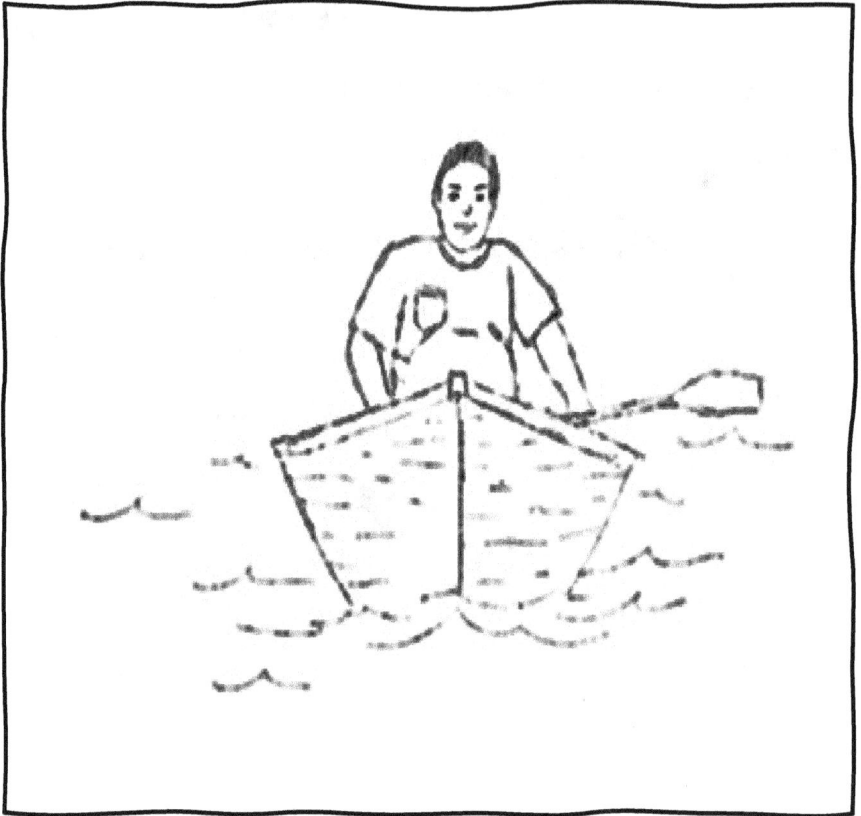

Carl worked there for so long that even
management felt like family. Retirement was just
around the corner and Carl couldn't wait. One day
one of Carl's bosses came up to him and asked

to see him in the office. His co-workers did NOT waste the opportunity to chant, "OHHHHH Carl is in trouble!!!" as he walked to the office. That's family for ya.

Once in the office, the manager explained why he called him in. "I know retirement is right around the corner for you." "Yep 6 months out," Carl bragged proudly. "That's awesome. Perfect timing. We have a program here that I want you to consider enrolling in. It's part of the retirement program and it's free of charge. Now I know you think you are ready for this big change, but it is just that—a big change. This program, called "Begin Again," goes through some of those changes and what you can expect right after retirement. It is a program loaded with tools and resources from fun to fear and how to handle both. It's built by retirees for future retirees. This will enable you to embrace what you have worked so hard for.

The End

As the summer went on, Mrs. R. found that her friends continued to share more stories of loved ones, mostly men and the struggles they deal with. These stories caused her to continue with her mission. She continued with a wonderful man named Olsen.

Book 7, Olsen
Part 1, The Struggle

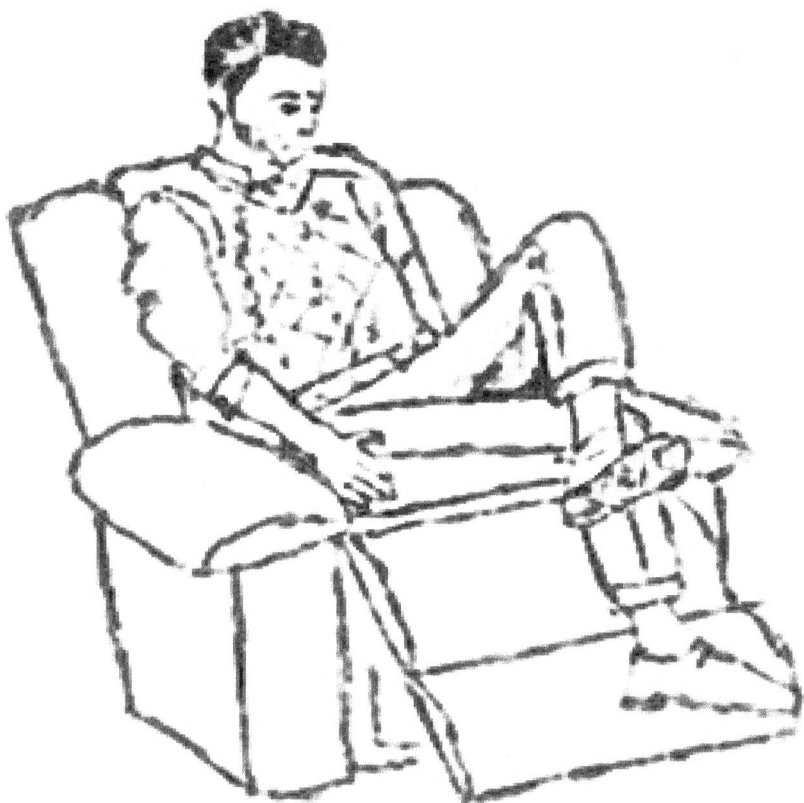

Once upon a time there was a man named Olsen. Olsen was the town's cobbler and oh what a cobbler he was. Not only did he have the dressiest men's shoe store in town, but he also knew how to keep any shoe looking its best. It was truly an art that Olsen was proud of. One reason why he was so proud was because he had inherited the shop from his father who had established quite the name in the community and beyond.

At first Olsen wasn't interested in running his dad's shop. Olsen wanted to pursue music, and so he did. He went on to get two music degrees from the most prestigious music school in the country.

Following his graduation, he enjoyed a plentiful career in the music industry teaching music at a university. But through time, his roots pulled him right back to his dad's shop. As his dad aged, he didn't want the legacy of the shop to diminish.

Olsen moved back to the community where he grew up, the very community he once longed to move far away from, and as his dad joyfully looked on, Olsen took over the reins. After a few very meaningful years, Olsen's father passed away. Olsen knew that the decision to move back was the best one he could have ever made. He knew that his father passed with happiness and contentment in his heart. The true meaning of rest in peace.

Olsen continued to grow the shop. Men came from all around in the search for fine shoes and to bring in their repairs as well. No one appreciated a good wingtip like Olsen.

Then one day, Olsen went "insane." He simply lost his mind. He didn't go into the shop. He just stayed at home. It was like a switch went off. He was kind, and pleasant, almost childlike at times. He could drive, and continued to go to the local gym, but he just wasn't Olsen anymore. With no family support, the community looked on with concern and compassion. Olsen's store just sat, closed and dark. Where did Olsen go?

Mrs. R. thought and thought about Olsen. She pondered about how different things could have been for him with just a few changes in his destiny. "AHA!" Mrs. R. exclaimed, "Here is your wish."

Part 2, The Wish

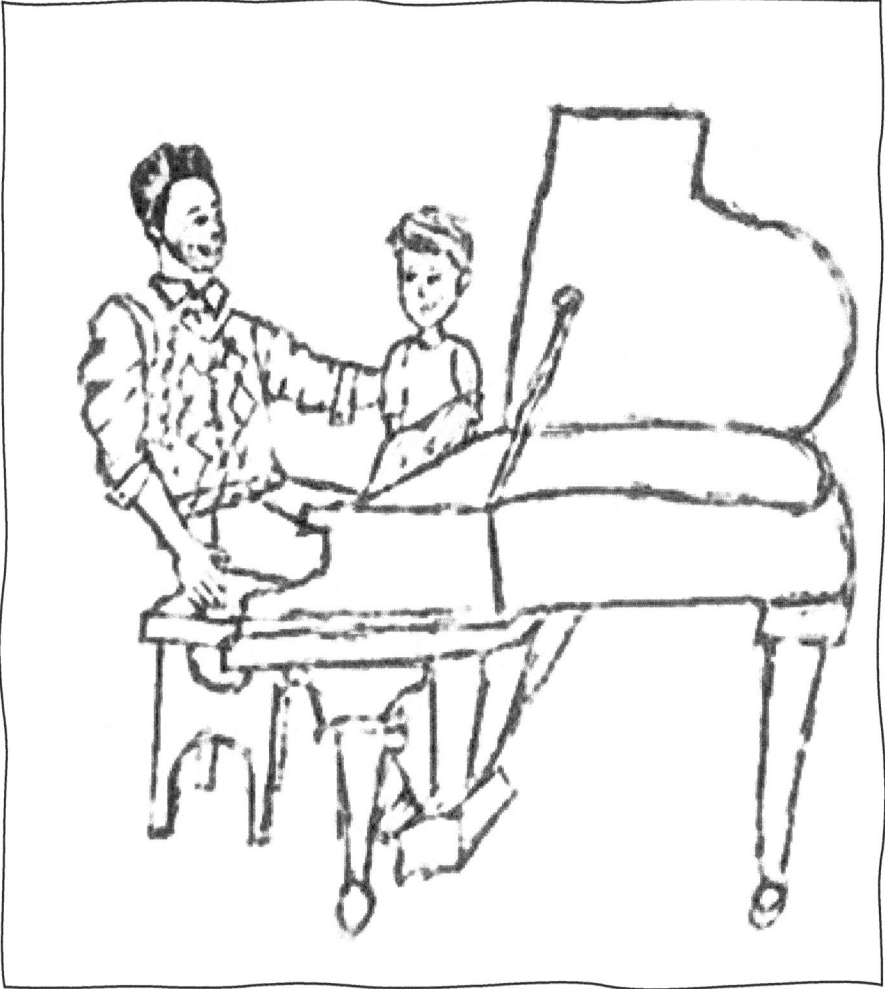

For years, the owners of the town shops

looked out for each other. They shared clients,

town gossip and good times. When Olsen didn't

show up to open his shop, the town barber knew something was up. He went to Olsen's house and found him sulking in his living room. He didn't want to talk, he hadn't gotten ready for his day, and he looked absolutely horrible. The barber called 911 and had an ambulance take Olsen to the hospital.

After extensive mental and physical therapy, Olsen realized that he wasn't alone in this experience. Other men sometimes face the same challenges that he felt. That realization alone made him feel better. With time, Olsen was able to recover and get back to his family's legacy. But he did make one change. He added on to the original building his very own music shop/studio. Part of what was missing in his life was music. With this addition he was able to have the best of both worlds!

The End

Being in education, Mrs. R. has seen her fair share of troubled boys. Each one would make her heart ache. She decided to write about a boy named Austin.

Book 8, Austin

Part 1, The Struggle

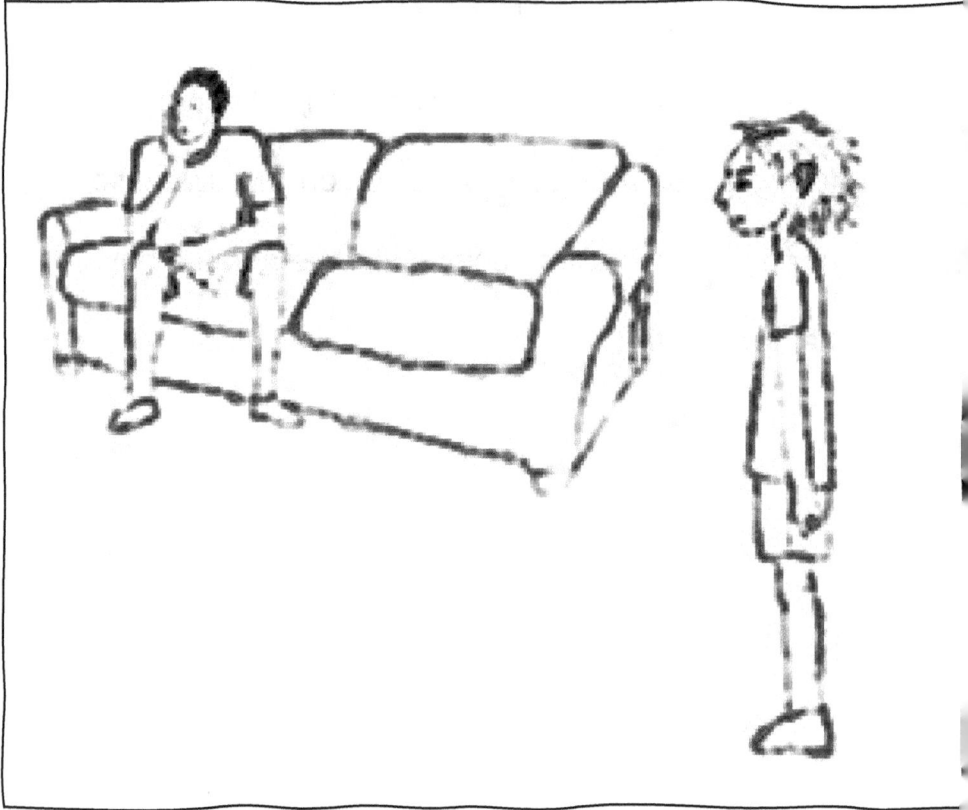

Once upon a time there was a little boy

named Austin. Austin was a magnet from the

minute he was born. He knew how to charm

anyone, man, woman or stranger with his big

brown eyes. He was a pleasant baby. He let

everyone know his needs, mostly food, and as

soon as he got what he wanted or needed, Austin

was happy once again.

As Austin grew, he and his dad had a very

special bond. It was clear they were of the same

blood. They seemed to understand each other

with no words needed. Right before his dad's

loving eyes, Austin was getting old enough to do

all the fun things in life such as riding a bike,

hiking, fishing and camping. Austin's dad couldn't

wait to share his vast knowledge with his son.

Austin looked up to his dad. He was

learning to be a strong and kind man just from

spending time with him. One weekend Austin and

his dad made plans to go to the lake and fish. But

when the day came, his dad didn't feel up to it. That was a surprise for Austin, but he tried to understand and went on to play with his neighborhood friends. "Maybe tomorrow," Austin said to his dad. "Maybe, son," his dad said with compassion.

But when tomorrow came, his dad said no again. "What's wrong Dad?" Austin asked. "I am fine son, just tired," was usually the answer. Austin's dad tried to gather the energy and motivation he needed to spend time with Austin, but he just couldn't do it.

Austin missed his dad and was too young to know what was happening. He thought maybe his dad just didn't want to spend time with him anymore. He wondered what he had done wrong. Where did his dad go?

Mrs. R. was writing away when she got a visit from her son. He asked her what she had been up to and with delight, she shared her journey on this hidden society of men's health challenges that she had been writing about.

She asked if he had heard of any stories like some of the ones she shared with him. Her son said "Yes, I have and there is a condition that I have heard of. It's called Andropause."
"Andropause? I don't think I have ever heard of this," she said. "Truthfully I don't know much about it, just that it exists," said her son. "But it sure seems to match some of the issues that your friends are going through."

Well, that was enough of that. She turned off her researcher brain and activated her mom brain, feeling so happy to have a nice visit with her son.

After her son's visit, she went back to her stories, imagining how wonderful it would be if she could really help to make these changes come to life. She went back to her sweet character Austin and added in what her son taught her about this andropause.

"Okay Austin, there is NO way you need to feel like this. Let's make some changes."

Part 2, The Wish

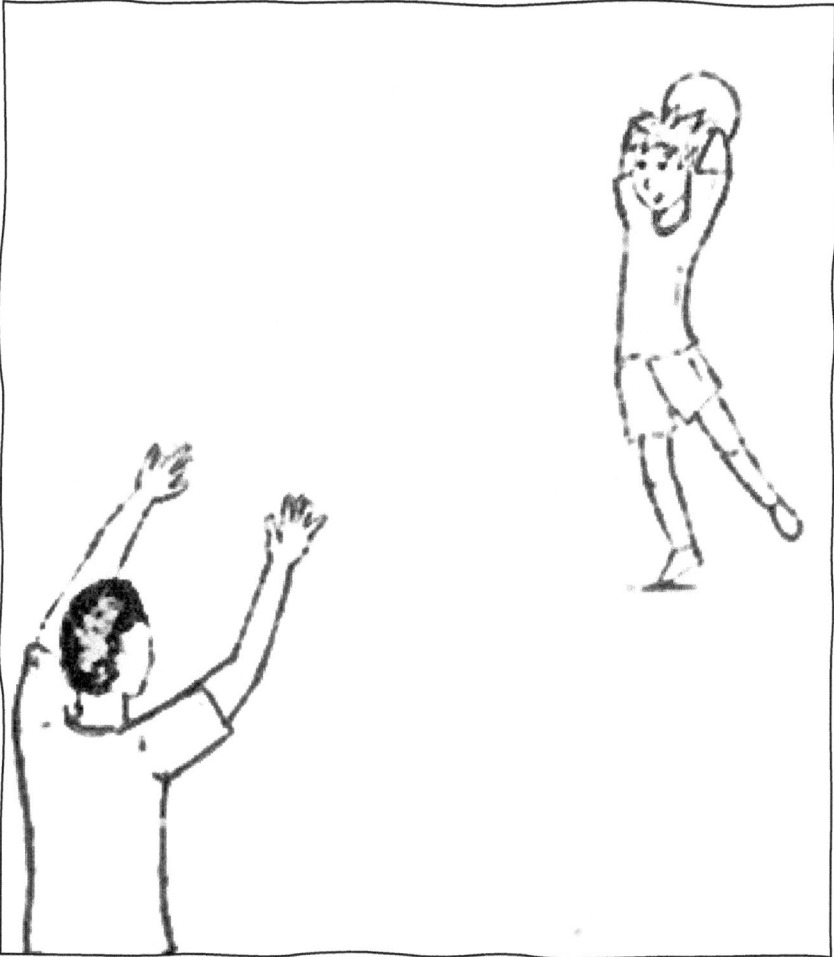

Austin told his mom about what he had

learned in school about this thing called

Andropause. He even showed the information

that was in his health book about how when boys get older, they can sometimes suffer a midlife type of condition that has many symptoms which last for various lengths of time. Austin's mom talked to his dad who had heard of it as well. He decided to get some tests done and put himself on the path toward healing. Soon, Austin and his dad were back together and closer than before. A bond was created that will never be destroyed.

The End

That's better Austin. She continued to weave this new term 'Andropause' into her writings. "Now on to my sweet Abraham."

Book 9, Abraham
Part 1, The Struggle

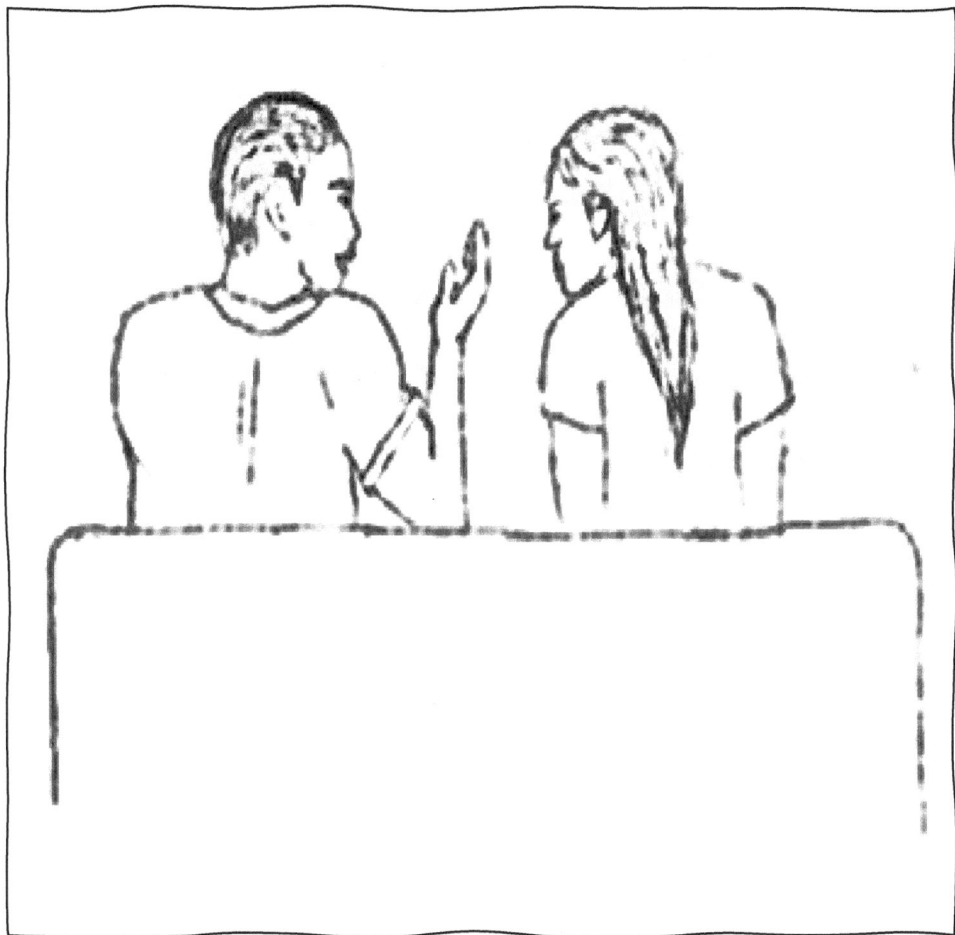

Once upon a time there was a man named Abraham. As if straight from the Bible, everyone loved Abraham. As a child, he was angel-like in his behavior. He always seemed older than his chronological age. Abraham was a kind and loving boy. Though a bit quiet in school, he was friends with everyone and everyone was his friend. Abraham was one of those people that if you knew him, you stayed in touch with him.

Over the years he and his childhood friends became lifelong buddies. He even went to college with some of them and stayed in touch with those who went on to trade schools and other callings from life.

Abraham graduated college, got married, had three children and a promising career. In his 40s Abraham was promoted to one of the highest positions at work. After years of striving to do his best, he was rewarded and rewarded with abundance.

For the first year after his new promotion, it was a dream job. But slowly Abraham started feeling differently about life. His work was great, the family was good, but the stresses of life seemed to get the best of Abraham. The little things in life that can become annoying seemed to irritate Abraham more than ever. He was still able to function at work but not with the same vigor that he had before. Through time, Abraham was able to re-establish a routine that kept him satisfied. He even felt like his old self from time to time.

Several years passed and the elders in his family started having medical issues. They were getting older and experiencing the things that so many people face with age. This brought some new challenges to Abraham and his wife. Serious decisions had to be made.

At first these life transitions seemed manageable. But after a while, the things that Abraham had to manage about his loved ones started consuming him. Instead of feeling younger and stronger and more capable than his aging family, he started to feel weak and overwhelmed again. Much in the same way that he felt when he got his promotion. He really couldn't believe it. He was so upset with himself. This was a time when he needed to feel his strongest, yet he felt that familiar wave come across him. WHY? Just like before, at first, he thought it would pass with some rest. But its persistence proved otherwise.

What was different this time was Abraham's frustration with the same feeling as before. How could he be going through this again? He was so disgusted that he even thought of taking his own life to simplify the lives of his loved ones. That was his mindset. Where did Abraham go, again?

"Come on Abraham, Let's see what we can do for you," Mrs. R. thought.

Part 2, The Wish

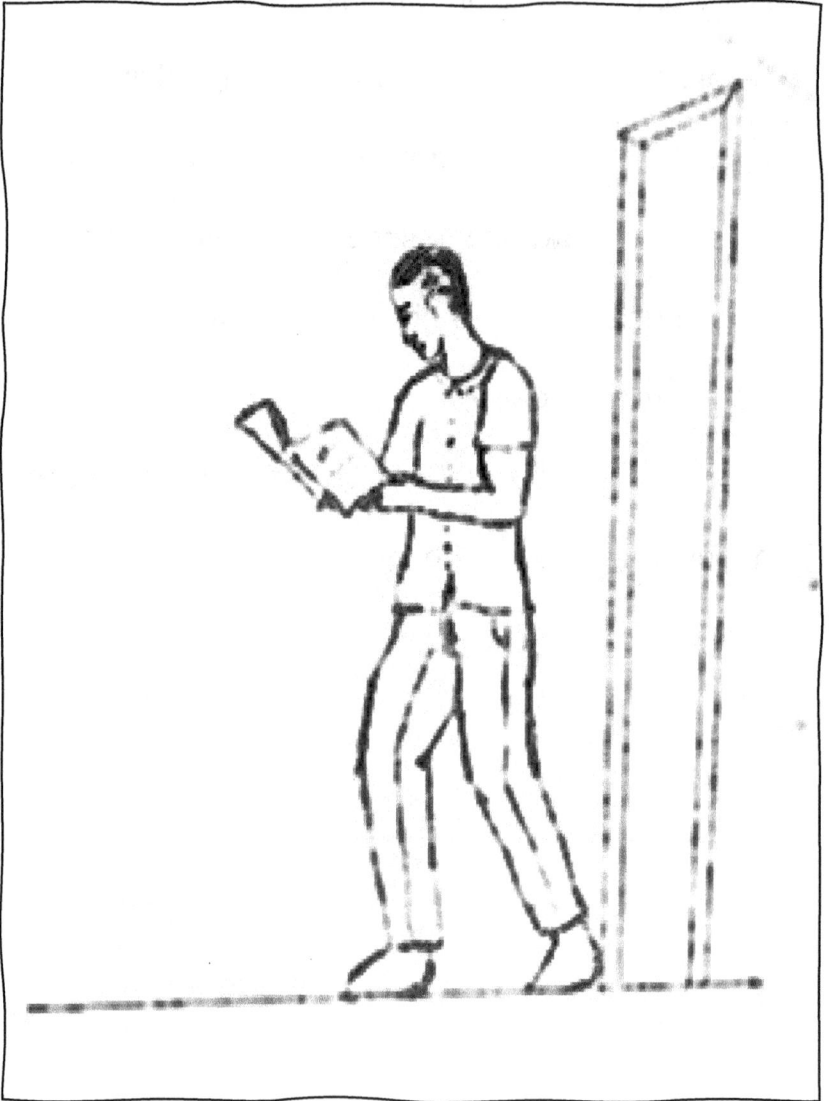

When Abraham started feeling those same feelings of anxiety as he did before, he finally decided to go to the doctor.

He admitted that he had these symptoms about ten years earlier. The doctor was quiet. He handed him a booklet called *Andropause, Before, During and After* and said "This was most likely what you were going through 10 years ago, and now it may be what's causing these feelings once again. At any rate, there are a lot of studies and research on the topic. We will get you feeling better."

The End

One afternoon Mrs. R. was writing away when she got a visit from her neighbor. It's always a pleasant time when her neighbor comes to visit.

It forces her to take a much-needed break from her project and enjoy some good conversation.

Her neighbor was curious about all this writing he had seen her doing on her back porch. She explained her passion project to him. He said, "Hey, I have a scenario for you." That gave Mrs. R. the idea for her next Tiny Book.

Book 10, Mr. No One
Part 1, The Struggle

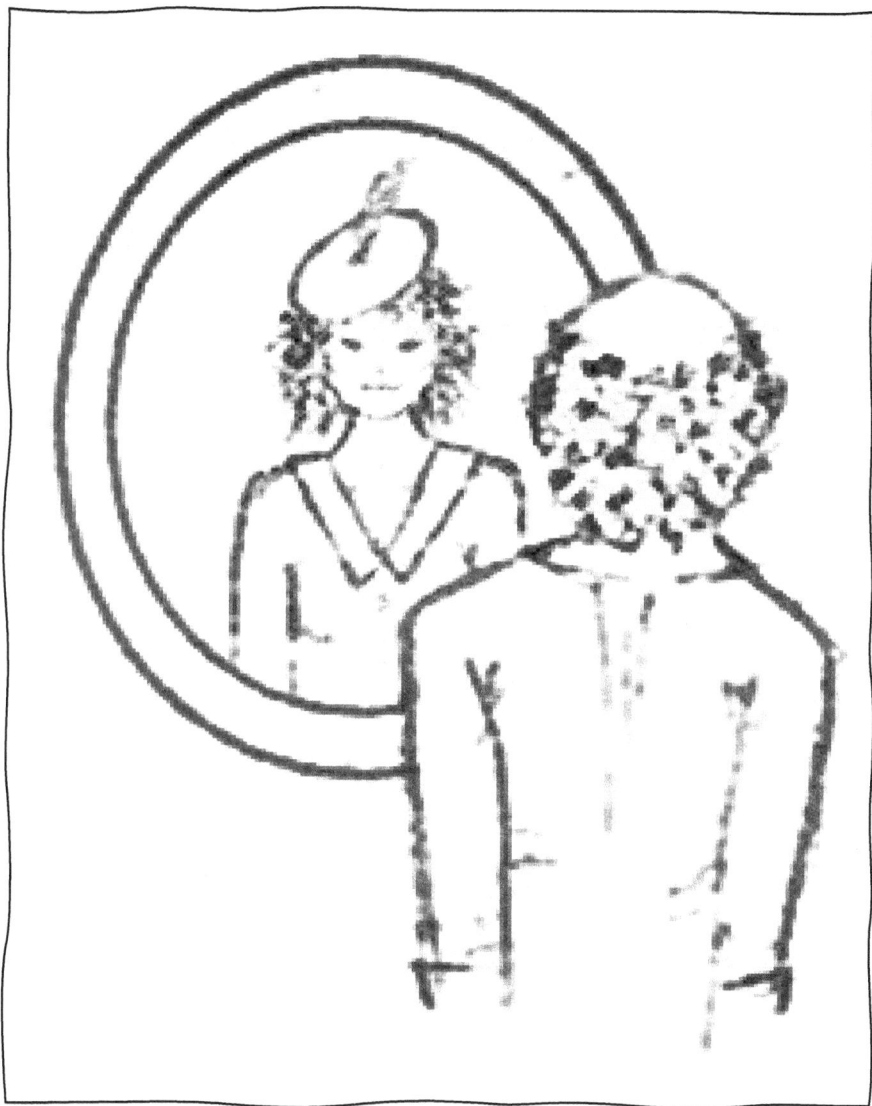

Once upon a time there was a man named Mr. No One. That was the name he would give anyone who asked him. "My name? My name is Mr. No One." And then he would shuffle off with the scowl on his face that never seemed to leave.

One day a young couple stopped in one of the restaurants that Mr. No One occasionally patronized for coffee. The young couple didn't know Mr. No One.

As the young man went to sit down, he noticed a wallet under the table. He reached down, picked it up and promptly gave it to the waitress, whose name was Sara.

Sara opened the wallet to see whose it was so they could find a way to contact the owner. As soon as Sara opened it, she saw a driver's license. She knew that face as if it were her own. It was Mr. No One, a man she knew only as Bill.

As Sara looked at the license, she couldn't help but notice the photo taped to the right of Bill's license. It was a beautiful woman, in a very old setting as if the photo was taken at one of those vintage photo shops that have all the old clothes, boas and such. At the bottom of the photo was the name "Ruby." That name perfectly matched the look of this striking woman.

The police station wasn't far away from the restaurant and since Sara was at the end of her shift, she simply walked over to the station to turn in the wallet and see if anyone knew how to reach Mr. No One.

She was greeted by the Chief of Police who knew Mr. No One well. Sara and the Chief exchanged some brief conversation, and at the end Sara asked if he knew anything about Mr. No One. She mentioned the photo of the beautiful woman that is alongside the driver's license. Sara asked if she may be a relative or someone they could reach out to. The Chief, with concern, said, "That's not a relative, that's Bill."

The Chief went on to explain that Bill was the most beautiful drag queen anyone could imagine. She won countless beauty contests and was well respected in the community of transgenders.

Bill never felt truly alive without Ruby. Ruby even had her own bedroom in his humble apartment. This bedroom wasn't just any bedroom. It was a bedroom extraordinaire. As soon as Bill opened the door to that room, he felt free. He felt like who he was supposed to be.

The room was styled after the traditional ornate wall and window coverings of the early 1900's. The bed was made of mahogany with intricate carvings on the four posters and headboard. The room had a sitting area for reading and listening to music. Ruby's closet was full of hand sewn gowns straight out of the early days with corsets and big bows, satin and velvet. The gowns were custom made just for Ruby. Who made them? Bill.

But perhaps Ruby's most prized possession was her cello. She was a concert cellist. She wrote a lot of her own music which was greatly inspired by the works of composer

Richard Strauss because of the playful and sometimes whimsical approach to his work. Ruby won several awards in the talent portion of the shows she entered.

As Bill got older, he found it harder and harder to be who he truly felt he was inside. His body started fighting him more and more and the beauty he was so proud and happy about started slipping away.

The pressures of the talent show business started taking over Bill's brain. Compiling that with his aging male body, Bill broke. He felt he could no longer be who he really was. His arthritis stopped him from sewing or playing the cello so he became no one, according to him.

Bill became a recluse of sorts. He knew he had to mourn his beloved Ruby. Piece by piece, wig by wig, he packed Ruby away in boxes, took them to a local vintage clothing studio and donated them. He took Ruby's cello and donated it to a local university. After he got all her belongings out of that room, he closed the door and never entered it again. Bill never recovered from losing such a huge part of who he was. Many feel that is what drove him insane. He continued to battle mental and physical issues.

"Come on Mr. No One, Ruby just can't disappear like that!" Mrs. R. brought Ruby right back!

Part 2, The Wish

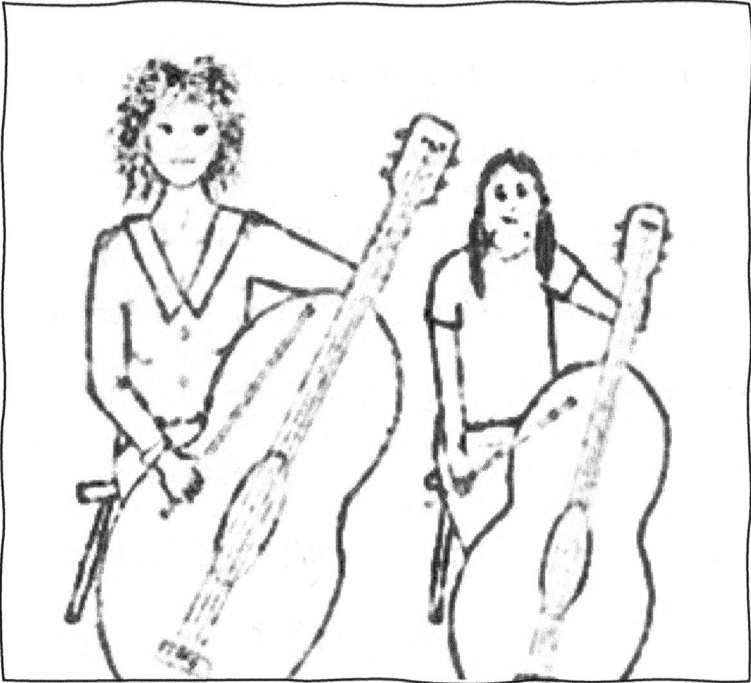

One of the important aspects of the

transgender community is that they have several

support groups to help and guide individuals who

may need medical or psychological resources. As

Bill got older, he was able to learn skills that

helped him understand who he was as a human

being. This made the aging process much more understandable, and he was able to prepare himself for his future, personally and professionally.

Ruby's beauty never really aged, because it came from deep inside her soul. Bill recognized that even though he and Ruby were changing, he learned to become at peace with it thanks to services available for people going through the same thing.

As for Ruby, she became an icon and someone that others looked up to in a world that at times is very uncertain and untraveled, but Ruby led the way!

The End

Wow, what a summer it was for Mrs. R. Before she knew it the curriculum for her classes was due and she was a bit behind her usual schedule.

She couldn't stop thinking about what her son had said about Andropause. In all her years of teaching, there has always been such a strong emphasis on what girls go through as they become women. They have very complex changes, that is for sure. With boys however, what she remembers teaching is that their voices change, they may get acne, an Adams apple becomes more prominent, they get body hair, and feel overall awkwardness. She doesn't remember ever teaching anything about complications that can arise as men age. Is it possible that men have a midlife change that leans more toward mental, emotional effects than people realize? Most of what she has ever learned about men is that if they have a midlife crisis that means that they will probably buy some sort of sports car or something. There are several commercials on TV about loss of sex drive but nothing that truly captures all the facets that may make up what men truly go through as they mature.

Mrs. R. decided to do something quite bold. She decided to do some research and add to the curriculum which has been taught in much the same way for years and years. She wanted to introduce her students to a more realistic life cycle of how men age and provide as many resources as possible for all students, friends, and associates. It wasn't easy making curriculum changes, but Mrs. R. didn't need easy.

After many meetings with the school board and other officials, she was able to convince them to let her make these adjustments. This new curriculum addition helped both boys and girls understand that everyone experiences changes in their bodies, physically and emotionally. These changes vary in their complexities and can be felt at almost any age in one form or another. No feelings are to be taken lightly and you MUST reach out and seek help.

This curriculum change, and the stories she wrote inspired others to join in her cause toward helping this hidden society. A group of mothers formed an organization called The Mothers of Boys, also known as The Mob Squad.

This is an informal group providing proactive materials on male health for every age and every stage.

Another group created a program that Mrs. R. added to her own curriculum. It was a program called Work Athletic Training, also known as W.A.T, a program that focuses on coping with competition in the work force and how to handle office politics.

One student created a forum called "Menvisible," an anonymous posting site for boys and men to go on and write their feelings. With a few questions about age and family history, boys and men can go on and express the things they are going through, fears and concerns. The creator hopes that these collections will be used as data for research by physicians who will specialize on how to help those who now have found a way to reach out.

Mrs. R. taught for several more years and touched the lives of many, many students. Finally, it was time for Mrs. R. to sell her home and move where things would be a little easier. She moved into an assisted living community and enjoyed it very much.

One summer day, one of the nurses came to get Mrs. R. from the courtyard. She had two visitors. It was a bit rare for visitors to come around so she was anxious to see who it was. There, standing in the community room were two very handsome men. "Are you Mrs. R.?" one asked. "Yes," she said softly. "Well, we just want to tell you that you probably saved our father's life."

"Really? How so?" The older brother replied, "Our dad's doctor was one of your students years ago. When you taught him about the issues some men suffer from that often go undetected and understudied, he decided he wanted to specialize in men's health for his profession.

When our dad went to him, he was able to diagnose our father's symptoms and help our dad in ways that no other doctor was able to. We just want to thank you for doing all you could to help raise awareness. You helped more people than you will ever know. My family is so grateful to you."

These kind words moved Mrs. R. to tears. For them to take the time to come to the center and talk with her was the kindest thing that had happened to her in a long, long time.

"I cannot express how much it means that you came here to share this beautiful story with me. What is your dad's name?" The younger brother said, "His name is Tiny."

They chatted a little more and exchanged goodbyes. As Mrs. R. watched the men walk away, she realized all these years later that she had never written the "Wish" story for Tiny. But it seemed she didn't have to. Life wrote it for her.

Her efforts to bring awareness had really come to fruition. Her "Wishes" were coming true. When she wrote these stories, each filled with love, sorrow, compassion and hope, she ended every one with "The End." But those two boys validated something that Mrs. R. had longed to feel. They made her realize that thanks to all her

efforts and not the end. It's only just…

The Beginning.

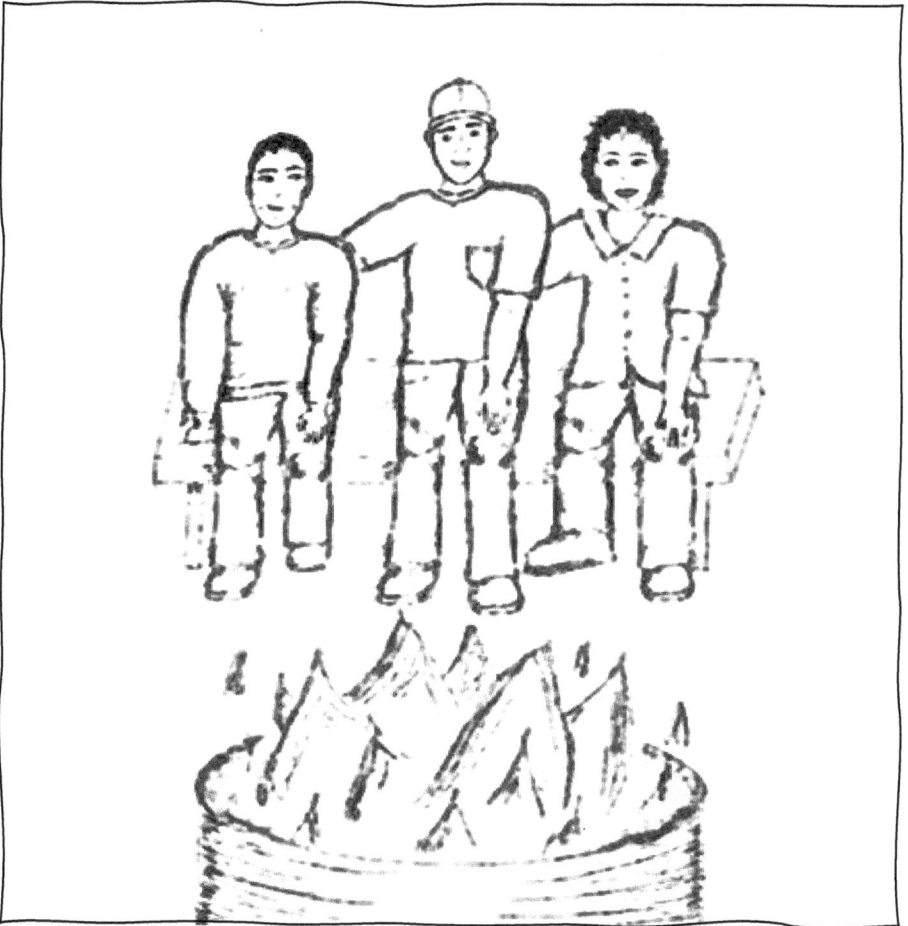

Andropause is a real condition. If you can relate to anything in this book, please tell someone. Reach out to a loved one, a friend, your doctor, just reach out. People can and will help you.

About the Authors, Michelle Swogger and the J Team

I call meetings with them. Does anyone else do that with their angels?

I'm blessed to live near a church where I go quite often to walk laps in the parking lot. It's a popular gathering spot for my angels. Years ago, when I lost so many loved ones, in what seemed like a very short time span, I started talking to them as a group.

I call the group Team J. Team J includes several of my loved ones from parents to life mentors who molded me into who I am today. I know each of them added their thoughts to the book. One angel in particular led the way. My angels clearly let me be the vessel to deliver this message.

My angels and I all have the same goal with this writing. To help others. We encourage you to read and share this with anyone you feel needs it. We thank you for reading and hope it brings a source of healing and inspiration.

I am pretty simple. My family comes first, pets included, followed by my careers–yes I have two careers and I love both of them. Through my family and the support from my work friends, I continue to learn that it is possible to find comfort and healing in places and experiences where I never thought I could. I have learned to keep my mind and heart open and observant. That has been the key to my own healing journey.

You may find me outside on my bike or in my healing hammock any chance I get. Two of my life's necessities for survival are sparkling water and chocolate.

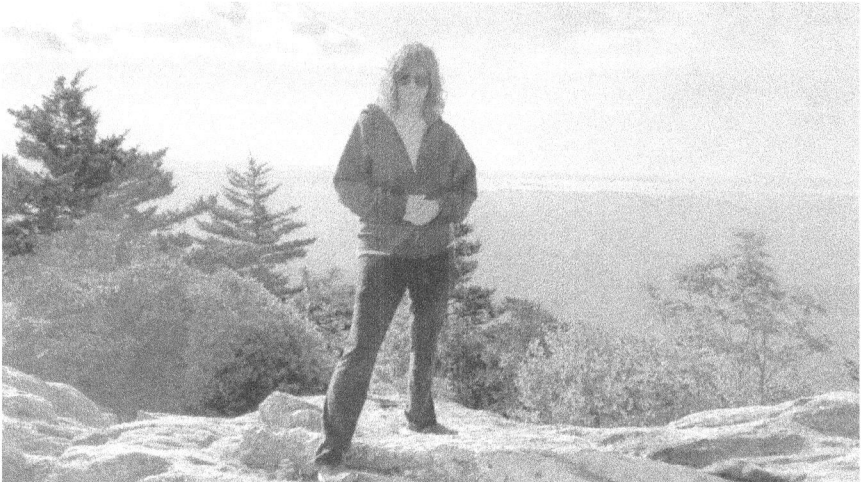

www.ingramcontent.com/pod-product-compliance
Lightning Source LLC
Chambersburg PA
CBHW072241290326
41934CB00008BB/1369

* 9 7 8 1 7 3 5 8 5 5 9 3 6 *